THE SCIENCE OF FAT LOSS

GENERAL TIPS FOR LOOSING WEIGHT

AHMED .R

Contents

CHAPTER ONE

INTRODUCTION

Due to its consequences for general health and well-being, fat loss has attracted a lot of attention in both scientific studies and popular culture. Anyone looking to improve their metabolic health and attain sustainable weight management must understand the science behind fat reduction. We will examine the fundamental ideas and workings of the science of fat reduction in this introduction, illuminating the physiological systems regulating energy balance, metabolism, and body composition.

The intricate interactions between physiological mechanisms that control energy balance, metabolism, and body composition are all part of the science underlying fat reduction. Here are some important ideas and working mechanisms:

Energy Balance: When the body uses up more energy than it takes in, a calorie deficit is created, which leads to fat loss. Reducing calorie intake (dietary modifications) and increasing calorie expenditure (exercise and physical activity) can be combined to create this deficit.

Metabolic Rate: The energy required by the body to sustain essential physiological processes like breathing, circulation, and cell repair while at rest is known as the basal metabolic rate, or BMR. Increasing BMR using exercises like high-intensity interval training (HIIT) and strength training might assist increase fat burning and speed up the burning of calories.

Macronutrient Balance: A key factor in fat loss is the diet's macronutrient balance, which includes proteins, fats, and carbohydrates. A diet rich in protein and fiber can minimize the loss of muscle mass during calorie restriction, maximize satiety, maintain lean muscle mass, and encourage fat loss.

Insulin Sensitivity: Insulin is a hormone that helps the body store excess glucose as fat and controls blood sugar levels. Enhancing fat loss and metabolic health can be achieved by increasing insulin sensitivity through dietary changes (such as cutting back on sugar and processed carbohydrates) and frequent exercise.

Hormonal Regulation: The regulation of hunger, metabolism, and fat storage is largely dependent on hormones including cortisol, ghrelin, leptin, and thyroid hormones. Fat loss efforts can be aided by balancing hormone levels through lifestyle interventions (such as getting enough sleep, managing stress, and eating a diet high in nutrients).

Timing of Nutrient Intake: The timing of nutrient intake, especially that of fats and carbohydrates, might affect metabolic reactions and fat loss. Techniques to improve fat oxidation, boost muscle repair, and optimize nutritional partitioning include carb cycling, intermittent fasting, and post-workout nutrition.

Genetic Factors: A person's metabolism, inclination to store fat, and reaction to food and exercise treatments can all be influenced by their genetic makeup. Even if genetics play a part, lifestyle choices like food and exercise still have a big impact on how much fat is lost.

Behavioral and Psychological Factors: The success of fat reduction is also influenced by behavioral factors, which include adhering to diet and exercise regimens, managing stress, getting enough sleep, and having social support. For long-term fat reduction maintenance, overcoming psychological obstacles and implementing sustainable lifestyle adjustments are essential.

People who are knowledgeable about the science underlying fat reduction are better able to make choices regarding their food, exercise regimen, and way of life. People can achieve long-term weight loss, improve metabolic health, and improve their general well-being by putting evidence-based techniques that target important physiological pathways into practice. But it's crucial to tackle fat loss methodically, consistently, and with an eye toward overall health rather than short fixes.

The science of fat reduction relies heavily on the ideas of metabolism and energy balance. This is how they connect to losing fat:

Metabolism: The intricate web of chemical processes that the body goes through to stay alive is referred to as metabolism. It involves two primary processes: anabolism, which uses energy to make new molecules, and catabolism, which breaks down molecules to release energy. The energy used at rest, or basal metabolic rate (BMR), and the total daily energy expenditure (TDEE), which combines BMR with the energy used for physical activity and the thermic impact of food (TEF), are the two further categories of metabolism.

Energy Balance: When there is a negative energy balance, or when the body uses more energy than it takes in, fat loss happens. This can be accomplished by cutting less on calories consumed, burning more calories through exercise, or doing both at once. On the other hand, as extra energy is stored as fat, a positive energy balance causes weight gain.

Caloric Deficit: People who want to lose weight usually try to maintain a caloric deficit, which is achieved by consuming less calories than they burn off over time. Fat loss results by forcing the body to burn fat that has been stored as fuel. To avoid metabolic adaptations and retain lean body mass, it's crucial to keep a moderate caloric deficit.

Macronutrient Composition: The diet's macronutrient composition has an impact on energy balance and metabolism. For instance, protein requires more energy to digest and metabolize than fats or carbs due to its higher thermic impact. By improving metabolism, maintaining lean muscle mass, and enhancing satiety, eating a sufficient amount of protein can aid in fat loss.

Exercise and Physical Activity: Both exercise and physical activity are essential for fat loss and energy balance. Resistance training, like weightlifting, and aerobic exercise, like jogging and cycling, can all boost fat reduction, raise energy expenditure, and improve metabolic health. Regular exercise can also boost BMR and help people maintain their weight over the long run.

Metabolic Adaptations: The body may change during times of calorie restriction in order to store energy and guard against malnutrition. A drop in body mass ratio (BMR), an increase in appetite and cravings, and a decrease in non-exercise activity thermogenesis (NEAT) are a few examples of these adaptations. Maintaining long-term weight loss requires an understanding of and ability to control these metabolic changes.

Individual Variability: Age, gender, heredity, body composition, and metabolic health are just a few of the variables that can cause substantial individual differences in metabolism and energy balance. Individual differences must be taken into consideration when developing tailored approaches to fat loss, as what works for one person may not work for another.

People can assist fat loss and enhance their general health by making educated decisions regarding their diet, exercise routine, and lifestyle choices by having a clear understanding of metabolism and energy balance. To achieve and sustain a healthy body composition over the long term, it is recommended to employ sustainable techniques that involve a moderate calorie deficit, giving priority to nutrient-dense foods, and engaging in regular physical exercise.

Adipose tissue, sometimes referred to as fat, is an essential part of the human body that performs a number of tasks including hormone regulation, energy storage, and insulation. There are various forms of fat, and each has unique properties and functions within the body. The primary forms of fat are as follows:

Adipose White Tissue (WAT):

Energy storage is the main purpose.

Location: Mainly found in visceral (the area surrounding organs) and subcutaneous (under the skin) depots.

Features include a solitary lipid vacuole, large lipid droplets, and a relatively low mitochondrial density.

Function: Stores extra energy as triglycerides. secretes cytokines and hormones that control inflammation and metabolism.

Adipose Brown Tissue (BAT):

The main purpose is thermogenesis, or the creation of heat.

Location: Mostly in little deposits near the spine, shoulders, and neck.

Features include a large number of tiny lipid droplets and a high expression of uncoupling protein 1 (UCP1) in the mitochondria.

CHAPTER TWO

Function: Produces heat by means of disconnected breathing, especially when exposed to low temperatures. aids in controlling energy expenditure and body temperature.

Adipose tissue, beige or brittle:

Thermogenesis, akin to that of brown adipose tissue, is the primary function.

Origin: Produced by white adipose tissue in reaction to specific stimuli (e.g., exercise, exposure to cold).

Features: Adipose tissue with in-between brown and white characteristics.

Function: Promotes energy expenditure and metabolic health by sharing some thermogenic characteristics with brown adipose tissue.

Subcutaneous Body Fat:

Location: Subcutaneous tissue, which is right beneath the skin.

Features: Offers structural support, cushioning, and insulation.

Function: Serves as an energy store and aids in controlling body temperature. In comparison to visceral fat, higher amounts of subcutaneous fat are linked to a lower risk of metabolic disorders.

Visceral Body Fat:

Location: In the abdominal cavity, surrounding internal organs.

Features: Releases inflammatory cytokines and fatty acids, and is metabolically active.

Function: Regulates metabolic health; nevertheless, excessive build-up is linked to a higher risk of metabolic illnesses such as type 2 diabetes, insulin resistance, cardiovascular disease, and others.

It's critical to comprehend the many forms of fat and how they work in the body in order to manage general health and lower the risk of chronic illnesses linked to dysfunctional adipose tissue. While some fats, such brown and beige adipose tissue, are good for the metabolism, too much visceral fat can lead to metabolic problems and an increased risk of disease. Therefore, it is essential to maintain metabolic health to promote a healthy balance of adipose tissue through lifestyle interventions such diet, exercise, and stress management.

The Mechanisms of Fat Loss

The body's intricate metabolic mechanisms come into play when there is a deficit in energy intake compared to energy expenditure, which is the physiology of fat loss. An outline of the physiology of fat loss is provided below:

Caloric Deficit: When the body experiences a negative energy balance, which happens when it uses more energy than it takes in, fat loss takes place. This can be accomplished by increasing physical activity, cutting back on calories, or doing both at once.

Lipolysis: The body uses a mechanism known as lipolysis to release stored fat from adipose tissue in reaction to a caloric shortage. The breakdown of triglycerides into fatty acids and glycerol is caused by hormone-sensitive lipase (HSL) enzymes, which are activated by hormones like glucagon, norepinephrine, and adrenaline. This process is known as lipolysis.

Fatty Acid Oxidation: After being liberated from adipose tissue, fatty acids are carried by the blood to organs including the heart, liver, and muscles, where they can be burned to provide energy. The body uses the mitochondria as its main site of fatty acid oxidation to break down fats into acetyl-CoA, which then enters the citric acid cycle to form ATP (adenosine triphosphate), the body's main energy source.

Ketogenesis: The liver uses a mechanism known as ketogenesis to transform certain fatty acids into ketone bodies in addition to oxidizing them. When glucose availability is restricted, as it is during fasting or carbohydrate restriction, ketones, such as acetoacetate and beta-hydroxybutyrate, can act as substitute fuel sources for tissues, including the heart, muscles, and brain.

Energy Expenditure: Losing fat also entails burning more energy overall, which is derived from physical activity thermogenesis (such as exercise), thermic effect of food (TEF), and basal metabolic rate (BMR). By generating a larger calorie deficit, increasing energy expenditure with exercises like high-intensity interval training (HIIT), strength training, and aerobic exercise might further improve fat loss.

Lean Body Mass Preservation: If exercise is not part of the weight loss plan or if the body does not get enough protein during times of calorie restriction, the body may also use lean body mass (muscle tissue) as fuel. Resistance exercise, avoiding too rapid weight loss, and maintaining an appropriate protein intake are all necessary to reduce muscle loss and preserve metabolic rate.

Hormonal Regulation: Important roles are played by hormones in controlling hunger, metabolism, and fat storage. These include insulin, leptin, ghrelin, cortisol, and thyroid hormones. Hormone fluctuations, especially those brought on by diet and exercise, might affect the results of fat loss and the health of the metabolism.

Individual Variability: Genetics, age, sex, body composition, metabolic health, and lifestyle choices can all have a significant impact on the rate and effectiveness of fat reduction. It's critical to take a customized approach to fat loss that considers personal preferences and variations.

All things considered, burning fat is a complicated physiological process that combines hormonal control, increased energy expenditure, metabolic adjustments, and calorie restriction. People can accomplish lasting weight loss and enhance their general health and well-being by comprehending the underlying physiology of fat loss and putting evidence-based strategies—such as calorie restriction, frequent exercise, adequate protein consumption, and lifestyle modifications into practice.

Techniques for Losing Fat

A multimodal strategy involving food adjustments, exercise, and lifestyle alterations is required to achieve fat loss. Here are a few successful fat-loss techniques:

Establish a Caloric Deficit: Losing weight happens when your body uses less calories than it takes in. Determine your daily energy requirements with a trustworthy formula or by speaking with a medical practitioner. Then, try to reduce your daily caloric intake by 500–750 calories by combining a healthier diet with more exercise.

Make Nutrient-Dense Foods a Priority: Give special attention to entire, nutrient-dense foods including fruits, vegetables, whole grains, lean meats, and healthy fats. Because of their high vitamin, mineral, and fiber content, these foods help lower calorie consumption while promoting fullness, controlling hunger hormones, and supporting general health.

Watch Portion Sizes: To prevent overindulging, keep an eye on portion sizes and engage in mindful eating. Measure your servings, use smaller plates, and chew carefully to learn how to determine when your meal is fully cooked.

At every meal, include protein. This will help you feel fuller and maintain your lean muscle mass as you lose weight. Every meal and snack should include a lean protein source, such as Greek yogurt, beans, poultry, fish, tofu, or tofu.

Refined carbs, added sugars, and processed meals should all be consumed in moderation as they can lead to overconsumption of calories and the accumulation of fat. Choose whole, minimally processed foods instead to help with metabolic health and weight loss.

Keep Yourself Hydrated: To maintain a healthy metabolism and to stay hydrated, sip lots of water throughout the day. Water is a crucial part of any fat loss diet because it can increase energy, decrease hunger, and improve fat burning.

Include Resistance Training: During fat reduction, maintaining lean muscle mass and raising metabolic rate require resistance training. Incorporate strength training activities on a biweekly or weekly basis, focusing on large muscular groups through complex movements like lunges, push-ups, deadlifts, and squats.

Incorporate Cardiovascular Exercise: Cardiovascular exercises, like cycling, swimming, walking, and jogging, can assist boost fat loss, increase calorie expenditure, and improve cardiovascular health. In addition to weight training, try to get in at least 150 minutes of moderate-intensity cardio or 75 minutes of vigorous-intensity cardio per week.

Put Sleep and Stress Management First: Give priority to getting enough sleep (seven to nine hours per night) and practicing stress-reduction methods like yoga, deep breathing, or meditation. Chronic stress and lack of sleep can interfere with hormone balance, increase hunger, and make it more difficult to lose weight.

Establish Achievable and Realistic Goals: Establish attainable goals for your fat reduction journey and monitor your advancement on a regular basis with tools like body composition analyses, progress images, and body measurements. Reward yourself for small victories along the way, and change course when necessary to keep moving in the direction of your objectives.

You may design a fat-loss plan that is sustainable, supports long-term success, improves metabolic health, and elevates your general well-being by implementing these ideas into your daily routine. For long-lasting outcomes, fat loss must be approached with patience, consistency, and an emphasis on a balanced diet and lifestyle choices.

Tracking Development and Modifications

The science of fat loss requires you to track your progress and make necessary modifications to make sure your efforts are sustainable and successful. Throughout your fat-loss journey, keep an eye on your progress and make the required adjustments with these crucial strategies:

Frequent Weigh-Ins: Weigh yourself on a regular basis, ideally at the same time of day and under comparable circumstances (for example, first thing in the morning before consuming any food or beverages). Monitoring your weight changes over time might give you important insight into how well your fat loss efforts are working.

CHAPTER THREE

Body Measurements: Monitor changes in body measurements including hip and waist circumferences as well as body fat percentage in addition to weight. Regularly measure these regions with a tape measure to track changes in your body's composition and the number of inches you've lost.

Progress Photos: To visually record changes in your body over time, take progress photos at regular intervals (e.g., every 4-6 weeks). Comparing side-by-side images might help you stay inspired on your weight loss journey by giving you a visual depiction of your progress.

Body Composition Analysis: To evaluate changes in body composition, including fat mass and lean body mass, think about utilizing techniques like skinfold calipers, bioelectrical impedance analysis (BIA), or dual-energy X-ray absorptiometry (DEXA) scans. More thorough insights into your development can be obtained from these techniques than from scale weight alone.

Monitoring Performance: Keep an eye out for gains in physical performance, such as increased stamina, strength, or athleticism. Even if scale weight doesn't change, increased strength or endurance during exercise can point to gains in muscle mass and metabolic health.

Dietary tracking: Use a smartphone app or a food journal to record the calories, macronutrients, and portion sizes of the food you eat each day. You can find areas for improvement in your eating habits and make sure you're keeping up a calorie deficit for fat loss by keeping an eye on your eating patterns.

Physical Activity Tracking: Use a pedometer, fitness tracker, or smartphone app to keep an eye on your level of physical activity. To make sure you're reaching your activity objectives and burning as many calories as possible, keep track of your steps taken, active minutes, and workout sessions.

Listen to Your Body: Throughout your fat reduction journey, pay attention to your body's signals regarding appetite, energy levels, mood, and general well-being. To better meet your body's demands, you may need to modify your calorie intake or nutrient timing if you're experiencing extreme weariness, hunger, or irritability.

Adjustments Based on Progress: Modify your food, exercise regimen, or lifestyle behaviors as needed in light of your progress and the input you receive from monitoring tools. This could include altering the number of calories you consume, the ratios of macronutrients, your exercise regimen, or adding more rest days as necessary.

Seek Professional Advice: If you're interested in losing weight and improving your nutrition, think about consulting with a registered dietitian, certified personal trainer, or other healthcare professional. A specialist can offer you individualized advice, accountability, and support to help you safely and successfully reach your fat loss objectives.

You can maximize your fat reduction efforts and attain long-lasting effects by routinely assessing your progress and making necessary adjustments based on feedback from your body and tracking devices. Recall that losing weight is a slow process that calls for perseverance, consistency, and an emphasis on long-term health and wellbeing.

Considering and Difficulties

It can be a difficult trip to lose weight, requiring careful consideration of many different aspects and the capacity to go over frequent roadblocks. The following are important factors and obstacles to remember before starting a fat loss journey:

Individual Differences: Each person is different from the next due to their varied body composition, metabolic rates, genetic predispositions, and lifestyle choices. Personalized fat loss plans that consider your unique needs, interests, and goals are crucial because what works for one person might not work for another.

Reasonable Expectations: Fat loss is a slow process that requires persistence, patience, and time to produce long-lasting effects. Establish reasonable objectives for yourself and recognize that big changes take time to manifest. Concentrate on moving forward gradually and acknowledge your little accomplishments as you go.

Healthy pace of Loss: To reduce muscle loss, metabolic adaptations, and adverse health impacts, aim for a moderate pace of fat reduction, usually 0.5–1% of body weight per week. Nutrient shortages, muscle loss, a slowed metabolic rate, and an elevated chance of gaining back lost weight can result with rapid weight loss.

Behavioral and Psychological Factors: It can be difficult to maintain long-term changes in eating patterns, exercise regimens, and lifestyle choices when trying to lose weight. Be aware of cravings brought on by stress, emotional eating, and other psychological obstacles that could prevent you from moving forward. Create coping mechanisms to handle stress, feelings, and triggers without eating to relieve yourself.

Adherence and Consistency: The secret to effective fat loss is consistency. Even on the days when you're not feeling inspired or have setbacks, make sure you continuously follow your diet and exercise plan. Set up routines and good behaviors that will help you achieve your fat loss objectives. Consistency is more important than perfection.

Setbacks and Plateaus: During your fat-loss journey, it's common to encounter setbacks and plateaus where your progress halts or you temporarily gain some weight back. Plateaus are not a reason to give up; rather, they are a chance to review your strategy, make changes, and remain dedicated to your objectives. Prioritize long-term trends over cyclical variations.

Social and Environmental Influences: Eating habits can be influenced by social contexts, peer pressure, and environmental cues, which can make it difficult to follow a diet plan for weight loss. Be ready to handle circumstances where eating out and other social occasions involve a lot of unhealthy food options. Make informed decisions, plan ahead, and use assertiveness when needed.

Metabolic Adaptations: In response to calorie restriction, the body may experience an increase in hunger and cravings, a decrease in metabolism, and an increase in energy conservation to stave off starving. Recognize the consequences of metabolic adaptations and take steps to counteract them, such as adding refeed days, modifying calorie intake, or cycling macronutrients.

Health and Safety: When trying to lose weight, put your health and safety first. Steer clear of fad diets, extremely low-calorie diets, and drastic dieting methods that promise quick fixes but may jeopardize your general health and nutritional status. Put your energy into changing your lifestyle in a way that will benefit both your long-term success and health.

Seeking Accountability and Support: Throughout your fat reduction journey, surround yourself with a network of friends, family, or online forums that can offer motivation, accountability, and encouragement. Think about collaborating with a qualified personal trainer, registered nutritionist, or other healthcare provider who can provide specialized advice and support catered to your needs.

You can navigate your fat loss path more skillfully and obtain long-lasting outcomes that improve your health, well-being, and quality of life by taking these aspects into account and taking proactive measures to overcome typical problems. Recall that losing weight is a journey rather than a destination, and concentrate on implementing long-term lifestyle adjustments that will enhance your happiness and long-term health.

summary

To sum up, the study of fat loss is a complex area that takes into account environmental, behavioral, and physiological variables that affect changes in body composition. A thorough strategy that takes into account individual differences, reasonable expectations, and potential roadblocks is necessary to achieve sustainable fat loss. A modest calorie deficit, a focus on nutrient-dense foods, frequent exercise, and treatment of behavioral and psychological issues can help people lose fat more effectively and enhance their metabolic health. A successful fat loss journey requires tracking results, making required adjustments, and getting encouragement from peers and professionals. Ultimately, long-term health, wellbeing, and a healthy relationship with food and body image are promoted by taking a balanced and sustainable approach to fat loss.

THE END

9 798320 800592